Frequently Asked Questions

# all about
# soy isoflavones
# & women's health

# VICTORIA DOLBY, MPH

*Victoria Dolby*

## AVERY PUBLISHING GROUP

Garden City Park • New York

The information contained in this book is based upon the research and personal and professional experiences of the author. It is not intended as a substitute for consulting with your physician or other health care provider. Any attempt to diagnose and treat an illness should be done under the direction of a health care professional.

The publisher does not advocate the use of any particular health care protocol, but believes the information in this book should be available to the public. The publisher and author are not responsible for any adverse effects or consequences resulting from the use of any of the suggestions, preparations, or procedures discussed in this book. Should the reader have any questions concerning the appropriateness of any procedure or preparation mentioned, the author and the publisher strongly suggest consulting a professional health care advisor.

Series cover designer: Eric Macaluso
Cover image courtesy of Barry Axelrod Studios

**Avery Publishing Group, Inc.**
120 Old Broadway, Garden City Park, NY 11040
1-800-548-5757 or visit us at www.averypublishing.com

ISBN: 0-89529-940-2

Printed in the United States of America

10 9 8 7 6 5 4 3 2 1

# Contents

*This book is dedicated to
the many important
women in my life—
especially my sisters,
Elizabeth and Carolyn.*

# Introduction

You've probably already heard some of the good news about soy: soy-rich diets are associated with the prevention of breast cancer, osteoporosis, heart disease, and even hot flashes during menopause. And scientists are still hard at work discovering even more health benefits of soy almost every day.

While soy can be a healthful addition to just about everyone's diet, if you're a woman, chances are even greater that you'll garner health benefits from soy. Soy plays a role in all of the greatest of women's health concerns: whether you are watchful of breast cancer down the road, facing menopause symptoms right now, or trying to head off the crippling effects of osteoporosis.

Phytoestrogens are a large part of the equation when it comes to the health benefits of soy. These plant compounds have gentle, safe, and highly beneficial hormonelike effects on the body. Soybeans contain a specific family of phytoestrogens called "isoflavones."

Ironically, the United States has become the largest producer of soybeans—yet instead of benefiting from the healthfulness of this bean, we export most of it. And what does stay here is either fed to livestock or processed into vegetable oil. It's time to change this and incorporate soy into our lives. The potential benefits are substantial.

Granted, soy won't help every health concern of women, but modern scientific research has confirmed many of the traditionally held beliefs about soy. Today, there is no question that soy has a lot to offer. Why not give it a try?

*All About Soy Isoflavones and Women's Health* starts out by answering your questions about what soy is, and detailing the health benefits associated with its various constituents. Subsequent chapters detail how these ingredients protect against cancer, menopause symptoms, osteoporosis, heart disease, diabetes, kidney problems, tinnitus, and other health conditions. Finally, there's a chapter explaining how to incorporate soy into your life: what forms it is available in and the supplement alternatives. There's even a glossary to help you understand new terms and a reference list of books you might explore for further information about soy and women's health. In short, *All About Soy Isoflavones and Women's Health* provides you with all the facts you need to confidently use soy to improve your health.

# 1.

# An Overview of Soy

You probably already have an inkling that soy is a "healthy" food. In this chapter, you'll discover that the soybean is virtually a pharmacy of health-enhancing ingredients. You'll learn why soy is a great addition to any diet, especially as a source of protein. Soy contains natural plantlike estrogens that have a number of important effects in the body—and this chapter will explain what these are. In these pages, you'll also get a sense of the history of soy as a health-promoting food.

## Q. What are soybeans?

**A.** Soybeans have traditionally been a food for both people and livestock. In some corners of the world, soybeans (and the many different foods made from soy) have served as an important component of the daily diet for thousands of years. Soy is a member of the legume family, and its main claim to nutritional fame has been as a source of protein. No longer. Today, soy is becoming increasingly known for a wider range of health benefits.

# Q. What can soy do for me?

**A.** It's almost easier to ask what soy "can't" do. The list of health benefits associated with soy—which will be explored throughout this book—include reducing the risk of breast cancer (and other cancers), heart disease, osteoporosis, menopause symptoms, diabetes, kidney problems, tinnitus, and many other chronic diseases. And scientists are continuing their exploration of this bean and report on potential new health links all the time. No, soy is not a panacea—but it does have impressive connections to maintaining and improving health, as you'll see in subsequent chapters.

# Q. Can soy serve as a source of protein in my diet?

**A.** There's a good reason that soy is referred to in China as the "meat without bones." In China and other Asian countries, soy provides up to 60 percent of the day's protein. And there's a good argument for Westerners to follow suit.

The protein from soybeans is generally equivalent to the protein in meat, dairy, and eggs. In fact, soy is one of the few plant foods that comes close to providing all of the essential amino acids (the building blocks of protein) in the proper amounts—although it does fall a little short in the amino acid methionine.

This slight shortfall in the methionine area is easily remedied by eating grain-based foods (such as rice, pasta, or bread) along with soy. Actually, most soy dishes already do this: from soy milk poured over cereal to soy burgers served on a bun.

Although the use of soy as a source of dietary protein is useful, that is not the most beneficial aspect of soy. In reality, most Western diets contain too much—not too little—protein, which means that additional sources of protein are unnecessary. It's better to use soy in replacement of other protein sources, such as beef or dairy products, that contain undesirable levels of saturated fat (a type of fat associated with an increased risk of heart disease and other health problems) and cholesterol.

But don't think of soy as just another source of protein. The real benefits of soy are the many phyto-nutrients—particularly phytoestrogens—it contains.

# Q. Can you tell me a little bit more about these phytoestrogens?

**A.** Phytoestrogens are a class of compounds found in plants, which include such substances as isoflavones, coumestans, and lignans. The chemical structures of these phytoestrogens are very similar to the estrogen made by the body or synthesized in a laboratory. This is why phytoestrogens can, in certain situations, act like the body's own estrogen. However, due to the slight difference between phytoestrogens and "real" estrogens, in some circumstances the use of phytoestrogens may produce antiestrogen effects. All in all, phytoestrogens make versatile contributions to health.

Phytoestrogens are found in fruits, vegetables, and whole grains. But the isoflavones are the most common form of phytoestrogens. And soy is the primary source of isoflavones in the human diet. Other legumes also contain isoflavones, although in less abundant amounts. Clover and alfalfa sprouts are the main source of coumestans, and flaxseed oil is the principal source of lignans. As a whole, dietary phytoestrogens are associated with a lower risk of heart disease, cancer, osteoporosis, and menopause symptoms.

# Q. Are there different types of isoflavones?

A. There are two predominant isoflavones found in soybeans: genistein and daidzein (although a third one, called glycitein, is also present in small amounts). Bacteria that normally reside in the digestive system are needed to convert the isoflavones as they occur in plants to a slightly different form that is usable by the human body.

# Q. Do any other plants contain isoflavones?

A. Soy is by far the primary source of isoflavones among commonly eaten foods in the diet. However, there are other plants that contain isoflavones in smaller quantities per serving than soy. These additional sources of isoflavones include red clover, alfalfa sprouts, split peas, pinto beans, garbanzo beans, lima beans, and several other legumes.

# Q. Besides isoflavones, are there any other beneficial constituents of soy?

**A.** Isoflavones have been in the center of the research spotlight, but there are many other soy constituents in the wings that also deserve attention. For instance, saponins are found in many different vegetables and legumes, including soy, and these compounds have many intriguing health benefits, including enhancing immune function, the prevention of certain cancers, and limiting the absorption of cholesterol.

Another interesting group of soy compounds that may be underrecognized are the phytosterols. Phytosterols bear a resemblance to cholesterol, but unlike the cholesterol found in animal foods, phytosterols from soy seem to block the absorption of the unhealthy animal cholesterol. Phytosterols also show a positive role in lowering the risk of colon cancer.

Protease inhibitors, yet another constituent in soybeans, block certain enzymes that otherwise contribute to cancer. For this reason, protease inhibitors have been shown in preliminary research to reduce the risk of cancer.

Another potential cancer-fighter in soy is phytic acid. Although phytic acid has the undesirable quality of binding with minerals, such as calcium and iron, in the intestine and preventing them from being absorbed, it also acts as an antioxidant to block the development of cancer. Phytic acid is found in many high-fiber foods, including soy.

## Q. What are lignans?

**A.** Lignans are another type of phytoestrogen. The most concentrated source of lignans is flaxseed oil, although small amounts of lignans are found in a wide variety of foods including legumes, whole grains, vegetables, and fruits. Actually, lignan levels are generally much higher in Westerners than levels of isoflavones, since soy is not frequently eaten, but several foods that provide small amounts of lignans are consumed regularly.

After being neglected for many years, lignans are now garnering a significant amount of research attention in terms of cancer and heart disease prevention.

## Q. What is ipriflavone?

**A.** Ipriflavone can be thought of as isoflavone's cousin. Aside from this link, the most exciting aspect of ipriflavone is its role in maintaining strong, healthy bones. Specifically, ipriflavone shows promise in the prevention and treatment of osteoporosis.

Ipriflavone, although not found in soy foods them-selves, does convert partially to the isoflavone daidzein. Synthetic ipriflavone is used, in some parts of the world (namely Europe and Japan), more as a pharmaceutical drug for the treatment of osteo-porosis than as a natural health product.

## Q. What about soy oil, is that healthful?

**A.** Soy oil is the main source of calories in the aver-age American diet (often hidden in processed and packaged foods). Although Americans are often admonished to reduce their intake of fats and oils, soy oil does offer the advantage of not containing cholesterol or saturated fat and being relatively rich in omega-3 fatty acids (the type also found in fish oils and linked to the prevention of heart disease). It would be far better for the health of this nation, however, if soy was used in a more wholesome form.

## Q. How did soy become part of the human diet?

**A.** While soy has been part of the Asian diet for nearly 5,000 years, it has only been cultivated and used in the West for about a century. Clearly, much of soy's history can be traced to Asia. The cultivation of soybeans was so important to Chinese culture that one emperor claimed soybeans as sacred.

For close to one thousand years, tofu has been a primary source of soybeans in the diet. But Chinese cooks have introduced many other ways to enjoy soy, including soy milk, tempeh, miso, and soy sauce.

Although soy hails from China, it also has a long history of consumption in Japan. Apparently, Buddhist monk missionaries brought tofu and other soy foods with them during their travels to Japan. Today, the Japanese consume more tofu than any other group of people in the world. For the sake of good health, it would be a good idea to follow this dietary example.

## Q. What are the benefits of an Asian-style diet?

**A.** Asian-style diets have plenty of benefits, particularly for women. Asian women suffer less frequently from cancer (of the breast, uterus, or ovaries) than do Western women. They also have fewer symptoms of menopause—particularly hot flashes. Soy seems to be the source of these benefits, at least according to epidemiological research that compares different populations. Additionally, research centered on the effects of soy in individual people reports the same benefits.

When Asian individuals relocate to a Western country, their risk of disease (such as cancer, heart disease, and osteoporosis) does not necessarily rise to the Western level, if they maintain a traditional diet. But disease risk rises hand-in-hand with a change to a Westernized diet. We can assume that the reverse is probably true: changing to an Asian-style diet (especially incorporating soy into the diet) can lower the risk of many chronic, degenerative diseases.

# 2.

# Soy Isoflavones: Unlocking Healing Secrets

Isoflavones are found in only a handful of plants, with soy being the richest source. In the plant, isoflavones appear to function primarily as antioxidants—protecting the plant from ultraviolet radiation and other sources of free radicals. When consumed, these isoflavones function as antioxidants and as phytoestrogens in the body. These two functions account for the majority of health benefits associated with a soy-rich diet. This chapter will detail exactly what the phytoestrogen and antioxidant activity of soy means for your health.

**Q. How was the phytoestrogen activity of isoflavones discovered?**

**A.** Plants have been suspected of containing their own estrogenlike compounds since the 1920s. During the 1940s, Australian sheepherders noticed that sheep fed on certain pastures of clover were plagued with infertility problems and showed signs of excessive estrogen levels. This animal-husbandry enigma was soon traced to the high levels of "estrogen mimickers" contained in the clover.

Research into these newly discovered plant estrogens during the 1950s and 1960s uncovered even more plants with weak estrogenic activity. And around this time the isoflavones in soy were determined to have estrogenlike activity.

## Q. Why does the body need estrogen?

**A.** Estrogen (the female sex hormone) actually plays several important roles in health. Estrogen is needed for fertility, sustaining a pregnancy, and breastfeeding, among other functions. Moreover, it appears that the estrogen levels typically found in women before menopause partially protect against heart disease and osteoporosis. But estrogen is not unilaterally beneficial. Too much estrogen in women can contribute to hormone-related cancers, such as breast and uterine cancers.

Estrogen circulating in the body (whether it was

made by the body itself or introduced artificially through such means as hormone replacement therapy) has a special affinity for certain tissues. The tissues that contain receptors that bind with estrogen are most common in the breasts, vagina, and uterus. When estrogen is bound to a receptor, it sends a message for that tissue to start growing. While this is healthy and natural during certain times of life (such as pregnancy), at other times it increases the risk of cancer. This is why a balanced amount of estrogen is best.

## Q. What are xenoestrogens?

**A.** There are many synthetic estrogenlike substances found in our modern environment. Pesticides, household chemicals, and many plastics serve as sources of dangerous xeno-, or foreign, estrogens. The problem with xenoestrogens start with the fact that they, like the body's own estrogen, bind with estrogen receptors and send a message to the cell to start growing, and even increase the number of estrogen receptors in the body. Furthermore, xenoestrogens prompt the body to release a chemical called "tumor growth factor." The end result is that xenoestrogens increase the risk of cancer (particularly breast cancer).

## Q. What's the relationship between xenoestrogens and phytoestrogens?

**A.** The natural plant estrogens—that is, the phytoestrogens—actually block the harmful effects of xenoestrogens. Phytoestrogens compete with both xenoestrogens and the body's natural estrogens. When phytoestrogens are present, they prevent other estrogens from attaching to estrogen receptors. Think of phytoestrogens as a broken key in a lock: the phytoestrogen does not open the lock (or in some cases it opens it slightly), but neither does it allow another estrogen "key" to operate the lock.

## Q. What happens after a person eats soybeans or another source of phytoestrogens?

**A.** Most of the isoflavones found in foods occur in a form that is not biologically active. Bacteria that normally inhabit the digestive system are needed to slightly alter the isoflavones before the body can use them.

Phytoestrogens then make their way from the digestive system into the bloodstream—and just about every cell of the body is able to take up at least some of these phytoestrogens. The reproductive tissues (including the breasts and reproductive organs) contain the greatest number of estrogen receptors, and for this reason are most likely to be affected by phytoestrogens.

When a phytoestrogen comes into contact with an estrogen receptor in the body, one of two things happens: either the phytoestrogen blocks the receptor (for an anti-estrogen effect), or it weakly activates it (for a weak estrogen effect). It is quite fortunate that isoflavones function as estrogen when the body's estrogen levels are low, yet seem to act as anti-estrogen when the body's estrogen levels are too high.

## Q. In addition to this phytoestrogen function, do the isoflavones also act as antioxidants?

**A.** Yes, isoflavones are also antioxidants, which help protect the body from free radicals. As you may already know, free radicals are highly reactive and destructive molecules found in air pollution, cigarette smoke, and ultraviolet radiation. Free radicals are even created inside the body during necessary processes, like breathing, transforming food into energy, or fighting an infection.

Over time, exposure to free radicals and the damage they cause contributes to dozens of diseases as well as premature aging. For instance, free-radical damage to low-density-lipoprotein cholesterol (considered to be the "bad" form of cholesterol) is an early step toward heart disease, DNA damaged by free radicals can lead to cancer, and proteins in the skin mangled by free radicals can appear as wrinkles.

In response to the danger posed by free radicals, the body had to develop a defense system, which took the form of antioxidants. Antioxidants neutralize free radicals or repair the damage caused by them. The body depends on many vitamins and minerals to act as antioxidants, such as vitamin C, vitamin E, beta-carotene, and selenium, but soy isoflavones also lend a hand.

The isoflavones in soy, especially genistein and daidzein, have antioxidant properties. Researchers at the Departments of Environmental Health Sciences, University of Alabama, Birmingham, tested the antioxidant abilities of soy isoflavones in animal cells. Genistein was the most powerful free-radical deactivator, although daidzein also had moderate free-radical blocking capability. This study also showed that genistein benefits the antioxidant defense system by increasing levels of other antioxidant enzymes. All told, isoflavones are potent free-radical fighters.

# 3.

# Soy and Cancer Prevention

Cancer is a scary disease, there's no question about that. There are a lot of ways that your diet affects your risk of developing cancer. Soy offers more than a glimmer of hope for preventing many types of cancer, especially the hormone-related cancers (breast, uterine, and prostate). Breast cancer is reaching epidemic proportions in some parts of the world. Yet in many Asian countries breast cancer is much less common. Soy is likely to be one of the factors keeping breast cancer rates low. This chapter will detail exactly how soy exerts this anti-cancer role.

## Q. What exactly is cancer?

**A.** Cancer is actually a group of diseases characterized by the uncontrolled growth and spread of abnormal cells. Normal, healthy cells are damaged and even destroyed when these abnormal cells invade surrounding tissues. Sometimes cancer cells travel through the blood and lymph fluids to other parts of the body, where they initiate new cancers. This ability to form secondary cancers is called metastasis.

There are two principal cancer stages: an initiation stage where the normal, healthy cell or its genetic code is altered and a promotion stage where the abnormal cell is encouraged to multiply. Both stages are necessary for cancer to develop. The initiation stage, caused by a mutagen (a substance that causes a cell to mutate) or carcinogen (a cancer-causing substance), happens quickly and frequently. The promotion stage, when a substance called a promoter is in contact with the abnormal cell, is more lengthy, allowing the slow growth of cancer to go undetected for decades. Cancer will not develop unless the cell exposed to a mutagen or carcinogen is subsequently in contact with something that will promote its growth.

## Q. What's the relationship between cancer and the diet?

**A.** Far from being a random disease, cancer (either its prevention or promotion) is intimately linked to non-genetic factors. In fact, diet, lifestyle, and the environment contribute to about three-quarters of all cancer cases.

Many substances in food instigate or encourage cancer. For example, food additives called nitrites, found in processed meats, such as bacon and bologna, are converted in the body into nitrosamines, which are potent carcinogens. Other dietary mutagens include aflatoxin (a mold that forms on peanuts), heavy metals such as lead, polychlorinated biphenyls (PCBs), and pesticides such as malathione and DDT. Alcohol does not initiate cancer, but it promotes the growth of existing abnormal cells. Examples of other suspected dietary promoters are saccharin, excess dietary fat, and excessive use of coffee or caffeine.

On the other hand, the diet also contains many anti-cancer substances. A diet low in fat but high in fiber, vitamin A, beta-carotene, vitamin C, vitamin E, selenium, and other nutrients inhibits the initiation and promotion of cancer. You probably won't be surprised to learn that soy falls into this category of anti-cancer foods.

# Q. How was soy's cancer connection uncovered?

**A.** Cancer researchers first became interested in soybeans when startling differences between cancer rates in Japan (and other Asian countries) and the United States were noted. In fact, rates of the hormone-dependent cancers (breast, ovary, endometrium, and prostate) can be as much as twenty times higher in the United States. And when Asian individuals immigrate to the United States, their cancer rates soon rise. This indicates that the initially low cancer rates were due to environmental (rather than genetic) factors. Soy is a leading contender for being the environmental factor that contributes to the low cancer rates in Asian countries.

## Q. What is it about soy that helps fight cancer?

**A.** When it comes to cancer prevention, the phytoestrogens are the business end of soy. As you'll recall, phytoestrogens compete with estrogens produced in the body or introduced from the environment (xenoestrogens) and prevent them from activating estrogen receptors. The cells that make up the breasts, uterus, and prostate gland are very sensitive to estrogen levels and are packed with estrogen receptors. A soy-rich diet provides just enough isoflavones to lessen the chances of developing hormone-related cancers, without the excessive amounts that could affect masculinity or reproduction. It's not surprising, then, that countries with a high intake of soy tend to have very low rates of hormone-influenced cancers.

The antioxidant abilities of the isoflavones cannot be discounted as a cancer-preventing tool used by the soybean. Genistein and daidzein disarm free radicals that would otherwise trigger cellular mutations. These isoflavones also boost levels of some of the body's own antioxidants.

Another weapon in soy's anticancer arsenal involves angiogenesis. Angiogenesis is the process of forming new blood vessels. Under normal circumstances, new blood vessels are formed only during limited times: ovulation, pregnancy, and wound healing. Angiogenesis steps into high gear when a cancerous tumor starts growing in the body. Large amounts of new blood vessels are needed to feed the enlarging tumor and to shuttle away its waste products. Isoflavones help to prevent this angiogenic process during cancer development.

# Q. Does soy have any other anti-cancer effects?

**A.** Isoflavones can prevent cancer in even more ways. Cancerous tumors are made up of undifferentiated cells. Differentiation is the process that tells a cell to be a heart cell, nerve cell, and so on. Without differentiation, a cell does not have a clearly defined "job description," which may result in uncontrolled cancerous growth. The isoflavones in soy prevent cancer by encouraging cancer cells to differentiate into normal, healthy cells.

It is also likely that the isoflavones arrest the spread of cancer by blocking an enzyme called tyrosine protein kinase, which cancerous cells use during their unhealthy, accelerated growth.

## Q. Can soy play a role after cancer has taken hold?

**A.** First, it must be noted that all of the research in this area is in a very preliminary stage. But scientists have noticed that certain tumors have a "multidrug-resistance gene" that acts as a pump within the cancer cells to expel anticancer drugs before they can eradicate the cancer. Greg Peterson, Ph.D., and Stephen Barnes, Ph.D., of the University of Alabama at Birmingham have demonstrated that genistein, " . . . and the isoflavones, in general, may be immune to the multidrug resistance phenomena." In effect, the isoflavones, in some difficult to treat cancer cases, may be one of the only treatments that the tumor is not able to resist. But again, this potential benefit of soy requires further research for confirmation.

## Q. Why do vegetarians tend to have lower rates of cancer?

**A.** Using soy foods in place of some or all of a diet's meat and dairy products (which contain substances that initiate or promote cancer) may explain some of the benefits of a vegetarian diet. Why? First, soybeans are packed with cancer-fighting antioxidants and phytoestrogens. Second, a vegetarian diet is much lower in total fat and saturated fat. Finally, substituting meat with soy-based dishes boosts fiber intake, and high-fiber diets have been shown to protect against several cancers, including breast and colon cancer.

Relax—you don't have to become a complete vegetarian to garner benefits. Replacing some servings of meat or dairy products with soy foods can give you some measure of protection. Even so, the more you base your diet on low-fat, high-fiber, soy-rich cuisine, the greater your cancer protection will be.

## Q. Why does breast cancer seem to be on the rise?

**A.** Researchers looking to answer this question have identified many risk factors for breast cancer—from a family history of breast disease to never having had children. But the most alarming theory is that the rise in breast cancer stems from increased exposure to xenoestrogens.

Although it's been known for a long time that estrogen promotes cancer cell growth, it wasn't until recently that xenoestrogens were known to do the same thing. Because both natural estrogens and xenoestrogens are fat soluble, they tend to accumulate where women have a lot of estrogen receptors and fat, such as the breasts.

Xenoestrogens increase the risk of breast cancer in several ways. First, they bond with estrogen receptors, just as the body's estrogen does. And after the xenoestrogen is attached to the receptor, the breast cells are encouraged to create new cells. Second, xenoestrogens trigger the body's release of a chemical called "tumor growth factor." Third, xenoestrogens can even increase the number of receptors, which allows more xenoestrogens to promote cancer.

# Q. How does soy help in the prevention of breast cancer?

**A.** The phytoestrogens in soy reduce the risk of breast cancer by usurping the xenoestrogens and taking up residence in the estrogen receptors themselves. The xenoestrogens are thereby rendered ineffectual.

Epidemiological research (research that compares disease rates among different groups of people) supports this theory. Japanese women, who have a very low risk of breast cancer, quickly assume the risks of an average American woman after moving to the United States and eating fewer servings of tofu and other soy foods. In addition, vegetarian women—who often include soy foods in their diets—are known to have a below-average incidence of breast cancer. It seems to follow that any American woman could lower her chances of becoming a breast-cancer victim by emulating a soy-based Japanese or vegetarian diet.

To further strengthen the link between soy and breast cancer, Dr. H. P. Lee, MFCM, at the Department of Community, Occupational, and Family Medicine, National University of Singapore, initiated a well-controlled study of 200 Chinese women diagnosed with breast cancer and 420 healthy women.

Frequent consumption of soy foods emerged as a protective dietary factor against breast cancer in these women. And the sooner protection starts—in the form of frequent servings of soy foods—the better chances are that breast cancer will be kept at bay.

## Q. Is there a "window of opportunity" for the greatest soy protection?

**A.** Even though breast-cancer rates start rising after menopause, diet and lifestyle choices prior to menopause (as far back as puberty) can often set the scene for breast cancer. For breast cancer, the benefits of soy (and soy isoflavones) are greatest when soy exposure occurs just before and during puberty. It is during this time that breast cells are changing—and soy protects the cells during this process. But it is never too late to reap the benefits of soy. No matter what your age, finding ways to add soy foods to your daily diet can benefit your health.

## Q. What about cancer of the endometrium?

**A.** Soy can also reduce the risk of cancer of the

endometrium (lining of the uterus). When the diets of 332 women who developed endometrial cancer were compared with those of 511 healthy women, some patterns emerged. Eating lots of soy products was associated with a lowered risk of developing endometrial cancer. Eating foods rich in vitamin A and vitamin C was also associated with a lower risk of developing this form of cancer.

## Q. Does soy have any effect on other cancers?

**A.** Soy has been found to protect against a wide range of cancers. For example, a study conducted in Japan found that people who included soy foods, such as tofu, in their diets had an 80-percent lower risk of developing rectal cancer compared with non-soy eaters. Similarly, soybeans were found to lower the risk of colon cancer by 40 percent.

Lung cancer may also be prevented by a high intake of soy foods. A study of Chinese women living in Hong Kong compared the risk of lung cancer and consumption of soy foods in 88 nonsmoking women and 137 control cases. After taking differences in age, number of children, and education into account, the researchers found that women eating tofu and other soy foods every day halved their risk of lung cancer compared to women who infrequently ate soy. Another Chinese study, this one involving approximately 1,500 people, reports that the more tofu in the diet, the lower the risk of lung cancer.

The startling differences between prostate-cancer rates in Japanese and American men was also a tip-off that dietary differences might be at work with this type of cancer. Men who eat tofu daily have one-third the risk of prostate cancer than men who only eat tofu weekly, research shows.

## Q. What about the conflicting evidence regarding soy and stomach cancer—is soy helpful or harmful?

**A.** Stomach cancer has been reported to be 40-percent less frequent in people consuming soy on a regular basis. However, not all of the research on soy in stomach cancer is positive. Studies that follow the use of soybeans, tofu, and soy milk generally find a protective effect against stomach cancer, but studies of miso (soybean paste used to make soup) are inconsistent. Some research indicates a protective effect from miso, while others have suggested an opposite effect.

This miso confusion may be explained by other ingredients in miso soup. Traditionally, miso soup is very salty, and salt has been linked to stomach cancer. Until further studies clarify the issue, it makes sense to focus on the other soy foods (tofu, soy milk, etc.) that show a strong preventive role in stomach cancer and to use miso only moderately.

# 4.

# From Menstruation to Menopause

The years surrounding menopause can be difficult for many women. The good news is that soy is a great option for women entering menopause. This chapter covers the many ways that soy's phytoestrogens alter hormone levels during menopause—and even how soy can be used as an alternative to hormone replacement therapy. The potential benefits of soy for endometriosis are also covered in this chapter.

## Q. How does soy affect the menstrual cycle?

**A.** As you may already know, estrogen levels rise and fall throughout the menstrual cycle. As levels peak, an egg is released from the ovary. And as levels drop (if no pregnancy has occurred), the lining of the uterus is expelled during menstruation.

Soy, a weak estrogen, can influence the menstrual cycle. Dr. Aedin Cassidy of the Dunn Clinical Nutrition Center in Cambridge, England and fellow researchers at the Children's Hospital Medical Center in Cincinnati investigated the extent to which soy foods alter menstruation.

Cassidy followed the diets of six healthy young women for four months. During the fifth month, each woman replaced part of her regular, daily meals with a serving of isoflavone-rich soy in the form of textured vegetable protein. Menstrual-cycle length, regularity, and date of ovulation continued to be monitored for three months after the addition of soy.

The soy diet provided 45 mg of isoflavones (the amount found in one cup of soy milk) daily. Despite this relatively modest soy intake, Cassidy found that hormone levels were altered and the menstrual cycle was lengthened. Women with longer cycles have lower lifelong cumulative exposure to estrogen, which in turn reduces their risk of breast cancer.

# Q. What happens in menopause?

A. The average American woman can expect to live one-third of her life after menopause, which usually begins at about age 50. (Although it is not uncommon for premenopausal symptoms to start occurring with increasing frequency about seven to ten years before this.) Menopause begins as the ovaries produce less and less estrogen. Without estrogen to stimulate ovulation, the menstrual periods cease.

The natural process of menopause comes with its share of symptoms, many of which can be traced back to hormonal changes. Some symptoms, such as vaginal dryness, result from the lack of estrogen. Others, such as hot flashes, are caused by more complex hormonal changes.

# Q. What is hormone replacement therapy?

**A.** Hormone replacement therapy (HRT) is the administration of estrogen combined with another hormone called progestin. Although this use of synthetic hormones is effective for reducing the frequency of hot flashes, it is associated with a slew of potential long-term side effects, including an increased risk of developing certain cancers.

For this reason, it is understandable that many menopausal women view HRT with a skeptical eye. Consequently, less than half of women eligible for HRT undergo it. Instead, more and more women are turning to natural diet and lifestyle therapies to manage their menopause symptoms.

## Q. Can soy isoflavones serve as an alternative to HRT?

**A.** Soy isoflavones are increasingly being considered as a viable alternative to HRT—particularly since soy doesn't have the risks of HRT, yet has the benefits of relieving certain symptoms of menopause and the bonus of lowering cholesterol, preventing osteoporosis, and lowering the risk of breast cancer, to boot. Phytoestrogens act similarly to synthetic estrogen contained in HRT in many ways. At the very least, phytoestrogens might reduce requirements for synthetic estrogens.

One of the early tip-offs to the potential benefits of phytoestrogens was the observation by researchers that very few Japanese women are plagued by menopause symptoms. As Herman Adlercreutz, M.D., of the Department of Clinical Chemistry, University of Helsinki, pointed out in a letter to the British journal *Lancet*: "High levels of isoflavonoid phyto-oestrogens may partly explain why hot flushes and other menopausal symptoms are so infrequent in Japanese women."

# Q. Is there any evidence that phytoestrogens can actually relieve menopause symptoms?

**A.** There sure is. A group of Australian researchers compared the ability of different phytoestrogens to alleviate the symptoms of menopause. Dr. A. L. Murkies and colleagues randomly divided 58 menopausal women who suffered from 14 hot flashes or more per week into two groups. Each set of women had their diets supplemented with either wheat flour (which contains the lignan form of phytoestrogens) or soy flour daily for three months. The wheat flour resulted in 25-percent fewer hot flashes, while the soy flour reduced hot flashes by an impressive 40 percent.

And that's not all. Italian researchers report that menopausal women who add soy protein to their diet gain relief from hot flashes. This double-blind clinical trial gave 40 women 60 grams of soy protein (providing 76 mg of isoflavones) each day for 12 weeks, while a control group of 39 women consumed a placebo protein powder. All of these women were suffering from severe hot flashes (at least seven incidents of moderate-to-severe hot flashes every 24 hours). On average, each woman reported 11 hot flashes every day before this study began.

The results for the women in the soy group were impressive: there was a 26-percent reduction in the daily number of hot flashes by the third week and a 45-percent reduction by the end of the twelfth week.

# Q. What is endometriosis?

**A.** Endometriosis occurs when some of the cells that normally line the inside of the uterus end up attached to the ovaries, cervix, appendix, bowel, and bladder. As menstruation approaches, these estrogen-sensitive cells respond by engorging with blood, which leads to pain and heavy bleeding. There are few treatment options, and the options that are available, such as hormone therapy or surgery, are unacceptable to many women.

# Q. Is soy a treatment option for endometriosis?

**A.** Soy isoflavones might be a natural alternative for women with endometriosis. Because endometriosis symptoms start when the cells respond to estrogen, lowering the estrogen levels helps prevent symptoms. When the isoflavones hook up to estrogen receptors, they prevent other sources of estrogen from activating the endometriosis cells. Although more research is needed in this area, preliminary indicators suggest that soy can provide at least a measure of relief.

# 5.

# Soy and Osteoporosis

More than 25 million Americans, four out of five of which are women, currently suffer from osteoporosis. Women are at greatest risk for developing osteoporosis because of their relatively small bones and the hormonal changes that accompany menopause. Soy, because of the phytoestrogens it contains, might alter the course of this damaging disease. This chapter also shares information about a substance called ipriflavone that has even more powerful anti-osteoporosis effects than soy itself.

## Q. What is osteoporosis?

**A.** Osteoporosis develops as bones become overly porous and brittle from a loss of calcium and other minerals. The end result is irreversible pain, loss of height, and bone fractures.

## Q. What is the relationship between estrogen levels and osteoporosis?

**A.** Low levels of estrogen (as occurs in the post-menopausal years) leads to an increased loss of calcium from the bones and to the development of osteoporosis. The longer estrogen levels are low (that is, the more years that have passed since menopause), the greater the risk of developing osteoporosis.

## Q. What is the conventional treatment for osteoporosis?

**A.** Hormone replacement therapy (HRT) is the most common drug treatment for osteoporosis. It assists in the prevention of bone loss in post-menopausal women, and 1,000 to 1,500 mg of calcium combined with hormone replacement therapy has been shown to be effective in the prevention of osteoporosis. However, the use of estrogen is controversial, as some studies have shown no benefits for its use in the treatment of osteoporosis. An additional problem is that HRT increases the risk of breast and uterine cancers.

## Q. Can soy take the place of HRT for osteoporosis prevention?

**A.** As your physician may have told you, HRT (undergone by many postmenopausal women) reduces the risk of osteoporosis in women after menopause. But phytoestrogens—by acting as weak estrogens—can have a similar effect. The advantage of using phytoestrogens in this way is the lower risk of adverse effects as compared with HRT. The unique thing about soy isoflavones is that they act selectively to build bone in menopausal women— like estrogen does—but in contrast to estrogen, the isoflavones don't promote breast or uterine cancer. In fact, they do quite the opposite and prevent cancer. And they are effective. When the effects of genistein were compared with the often-prescribed synthetic estrogen Premarin, genistein was shown to have similar effects in maintaining bone density, according to animal research.

## Q. What is the role of calcium in osteoporosis?

**A.** Osteoporosis may be a preventable disease— and adequate intake of calcium throughout life appears to be the key preventive step. During childhood and adolescence, calcium is crucial for the development of strong, dense bones. During the middle years, when calcium loss from bones exceeds calcium gain, calcium supplementation may slow the rate of bone loss. Finally, during and after menopause, calcium is essential to prevent the rapid bone loss associated with the advanced stages of osteoporosis.

The adult Recommended Dietary Allowance (RDA) for calcium of 800 mg per day may not be adequate to prevent osteoporosis, and it is recommended that premenopausal women consume 1,000 mg daily. Postmenopausal women who are not using HRT might require as much as 1,500 mg to 1,700 mg of calcium daily.

Calcium is slowly lost from the bones beginning at about age 30. So by the time a woman enters menopause, as much as one-third to two-thirds of her original bone tissue may have been lost. In addition, a poor diet before age 35 can result in smaller bones—with less calcium to lose before advanced stages of osteoporosis develop. To date, the best treatment for osteoporosis is prevention. And optimal calcium intake is a big part of any prevention program.

# Q. In addition to being a source of phytoestrogens, can soy prevent osteoporosis by supplying calcium?

**A.** Yes. Many soy foods are a source of calcium. A serving of tofu (one-quarter block)—when made from soy milk processed with calcium salts—provides 406 mg of calcium. Other soy foods, such as miso and tempeh, provide 92 mg and 77 mg of calcium per serving, respectively. And soy milk fortified with calcium is becoming increasingly common.

Another way in which soy foods fight against osteoporosis is by replacing some of the animal protein (meat, dairy, and eggs) in a diet. These animal proteins cause the body to lose up to 50-percent more calcium than the protein in soy.

# Q. What effect does ipriflavone have on osteoporosis?

**A.** Ipriflavone—a substance similar to isoflavones—is emerging as a new treatment for osteoporosis. Ipriflavone has been shown to increase bone mineral density, which makes bones more resistant to osteoporosis.

Knowledge of ipriflavone's role in preventing

osteoporosis goes back to animal studies conducted in the early 1970s. Continued research has confirmed its benefits, and ipriflavone is approved for the treatment of bone loss in Hungary, Italy, and Japan.

Maria Luisa Brandi, MD, PhD, of the University of Florence, Italy, reviewed the role of ipriflavone in the treatment of osteoporosis. Brandi found that although ipriflavone doesn't have a direct estrogen-like effect, it does, in other ways, increase the mineralization of bone.

Dr. Attila B. Kovás, a Hungarian researcher at the Clinical Development Group in Budapest, has also investigated the efficacy of ipriflavone in a yearlong double-blind study of 91 postmenopausal women. Again, ipriflavone was shown to have a favorable effect in treating osteoporosis. However, an interesting wrinkle emerged from this study. Kovás explains: "Although the ipriflavone was administered continuously for 12 months, the peak effect was seen after 6 months. . . . From a clinical point of view, it might be possible to achieve even better results with intermittent ipriflavone therapy."

Even more effective was a study that used a combination of ipriflavone and calcium supplements to prevent bone loss that occurs right after menopause.

The optimal dose appears to be 600 mg of ipriflavone for treating osteoporosis. On the whole, ipriflavone appears to be very promising as an alternative treatment for osteoporosis for women who either cannot use or choose not to use HRT.

# Q. How does ipriflavone work?

**A.** The way that ipriflavone prevents osteoporosis appears to be by blocking the resorption (disintegration) of bone. Alternatively, since one of the breakdown products of ipriflavone is the isoflavone daidzein, it is possible that the anti-osteoporotic benefits are related to this phytoestrogen.

# 6.

# Soy and Heart Health

**H**eart disease kills more Americans than any other disease. However, the simple soybean can go a long way to prevent it. Many women consider incorporating soy into their diets (or taking soy supplements) to gain relief from menopause symptoms or for breast cancer protection, but some added benefits for such women are lower cholesterol levels and less risk of heart disease.

**Q. Heart disease seems like such a "male" disease, why should women be concerned with it?**

**A.** When comparing men and women of all ages, women account for slightly more than half of all heart attacks. In fact, a woman is eleven times more likely to die from a heart attack than from breast cancer. Clearly, women are not immune against heart disease.

# Q. How are hormones connected to heart disease?

**A.** Actually, heart disease can be viewed as a hormone-dependent disease, since premenopausal women are somewhat protected from this disease, and heart disease rates in postmenopausal women rise to meet that of males. Estrogen provides this measure of protection against heart disease for women. After menopause, when estrogen levels decline markedly, high-density-lipoprotein (HDL) cholesterol (considered to be the "good," or beneficial, cholesterol) tends to decrease and LDL cholesterol (the "bad" cholesterol) tends to increase—thus promoting heart disease.

This accounts, in part, for why premenopausal women are at lower risk for heart disease and why HRT helps protect against heart disease in postmenopausal women. Perhaps phytoestrogens in soy can exert similar, beneficial effects—without the undesirable side effects of HRT.

# Q. How recent is the discovery that soy protects against heart disease?

**A.** The protection soy affords against heart disease

is far from a recent discovery. It is only the acknowl-edgment of this fact that is new. Back at the turn of the century, Russian scientists first noted that soy protein in the diets of laboratory animals kept cholesterol levels down. But it wasn't for another fifty years that soy protein diets were tested on human subjects—with the same results. Even when people have a moderately high intake of cholesterol, soy protein is able to keep cholesterol levels in check.

# Q. Do people who eat soy have a lower risk of heart disease?

**A.** One way that scientists try to figure out whether a certain style of eating has health merits is to compare the health status of people eating that diet with those who don't. In the case of soy, there was a study that compared soy intake in almost 5,000 men and women and then cross-checked this with their cholesterol levels. A significant trend emerged, which linked higher soy intakes with lower cholesterol levels.

The benefits that soy provides remained strong, even after the researchers controlled for other fac-tors known to influence cholesterol, including age, smoking, fat intake, and, for women, menopause.

The protein in soy was closely tied to its cholesterol-lowering ability.

## Q. But how effective is soy for controlling cholesterol?

A. There are no two ways about it, soy is a powerful way to keep cholesterol levels in check. Adding soy protein to the diet lowers heart disease risk by 20 to 30 percent, according to landmark research published in the *New England Journal of Medicine*. James W. Anderson, MD, an endocrinologist and nutritionist at the Veterans Affairs Medical Center and Department of Medicine, compiled this data by pooling together 38 controlled trials for reanalysis. Individually, each study was too small to show significant results, but taken as a whole, the findings would be more weighty. This type of study is known as a "meta-analysis."

Anderson found that a soy diet resulted in a drop in total cholesterol levels in 89 percent of the studies. Four studies did not show a significant decrease, but these included patients who already had low cholesterol levels. Overall, adding soy to the diet led to a 23.2 mg per deciliter drop in total cholesterol levels. Soy protein was found to lower LDL-cholesterol levels by approximately 13 percent (or 21. 7 mg per deciliter). HDL cholesterol was not significantly affected by soy protein, although the tendency was toward a beneficial increase. And eating just two or three servings of soy foods each day, such as by substituting soy milk for dairy milk and using tofu, is adequate to achieve these benefits.

# Q. How does soy do it?

**A.** The amino-acid profile of soy may explain how it lowers cholesterol levels, and in turn lowers the risk of heart disease. Every protein-rich food has a unique amino-acid profile, lower in some amino acids and higher in others. Soybeans are high in two amino acids: glycine and arginine. These amino acids lower insulin levels in the body and thus decrease the amount of cholesterol manufactured by the body. Conversely, animal proteins are high in the amino acid lysine, which *raises* insulin, and therefore, cholesterol levels.

The antioxidant isoflavones in soy are also important in preventing heart disease. Free radicals, highly reactive and unstable molecules, contribute to heart disease when they target LDL cholesterol. LDL cholesterol damaged by free radicals hastens the development of coronary heart disease. Fortunately, the body has a system for disarming free radicals and preventing them from damaging LDL cholesterol and other cells of the body. Vitamins C and E, beta-carotene, and selenium make up the core of the antioxidant defense system. But genistein and daidzein also play an antioxidant role in protecting LDL cholesterol and other parts of the body.

Preliminary research shows that soybean saponins lower cholesterol levels by either blocking the absorption or increasing the excretion of cholesterol from the body. Phytosterols, another substance in soy that resemble cholesterol, may also lower cholesterol levels. Phytosterols work by competing with dietary cholesterol for absorption.

Susan M. Potter of the University of Illinois at Urbana-Champaign recently evaluated the various methods by which soy lowers cholesterol. She found that soy protein seems to "pull" cholesterol from the body. In addition, she explained that some evidence indicates that a diet rich in soy alters hormone levels, especially thyroid hormones, in such a way that beneficially affects the production of cholesterol.

# 7.

# Soy and Other Health Concerns

Soy is a versatile way to maintain good health. There are many ways, in addition to those discussed in earlier chapters, that soy protects against disease. This chapter will outline the benefits of soy for diabetics and those with kidney disease, kidney stones, gallstones, tinnitus, and autoimmune disorders.

## Q. What connection does soy have with diabetes?

**A.** Soy was first recommended for use by diabetics back in 1910. In fact, this was the first time soy was associated with any type of health benefit. The original rationale for the potential connection between soy and improved symptoms was the low glycogen (carbohydrate) content of soy.

# Q. What goes wrong in a diabetic?

**A.** Normally, insulin (a hormone produced by the pancreas) is made in response to the level of sugar in the bloodstream. Carbohydrates are absorbed from the intestine into the bloodstream in the form of glucose and other simple sugars. This rise in blood sugar causes insulin to be secreted from the pancreas, which encourages the transportation of sugar from the blood into the cells. Insulin serves two purposes: it lowers blood sugar levels and increases the availability of sugar for normal cell functioning. Blood insulin levels return to pre-meal levels as the blood sugar levels also decrease.

Things happen differently in the diabetic. The rise in blood sugar after a meal either results in no insulin secretion from the pancreas or causes normal amounts to be secreted but the cells do not respond to the hormone. As a result, blood-sugar levels remain high; sugar spills into the urine; and complications may develop, such as eye disorders and circulation problems. In addition, the cells are starved for energy, so stored fat is broken down, raising the blood fat levels and increasing the diabetic's risk for developing cardiovascular disease.

# Q. How can soy help diabetes?

**A.** A diet higher in complex carbohydrates, such as whole-grain breads and cereals, vegetables, cooked dried beans and peas, potatoes, and other unrefined starches, rather than in protein and fat helps control diabetes. Fiber, especially soluble fiber (the kind in soy), helps the body handle changes in blood-sugar levels. A low-fiber meal is absorbed quickly into the blood and causes a surge in blood-sugar levels. In contrast, a high-fiber meal "gels" in the intestine, slowing down the absorption of food. This less severe rise in blood sugar is easier for a diabetic's body to deal with.

Additional research shows that when the diet is high in fiber, the cells are more sensitive to insulin and increase their number of insulin receptor sites. In addition, high-fiber diets are associated with less sugar in the urine, lower blood sugar levels, and lower insulin requirements.

Soy foods, such as whole soybeans, tofu, tempeh, and textured vegetable protein, provide a large amount of the soluble fiber found to benefit diabetes. Many diabetics decrease or even eliminate their need for insulin after changing to a high-fiber diet. The best results are seen in diabetics who are taking less than 30 units of insulin, in type II diabetics, and/or those who also lose weight (if they are overweight).

Hypoglycemia is a condition of abnormally low levels of blood sugar. Most cases occur in type I diabetics, after they take excessive blood-sugar-lowering drugs, miss a meal, or exercise excessively. This condition also occasionally develops in a non-diabetic whose pancreas simply produces too much insulin in response to rising blood sugar levels. In either case, symptoms of weakness, hunger, dizziness, and even coma develop. The soluble fiber in soy may help normalize blood sugar/insulin levels for hypoglycemics.

## Q. Does soy aid in the prevention of kidney disease?

**A.** A lifelong diet of animal protein can be damaging to the kidneys, since the kidneys have to filter the byproducts of animal protein. In contrast, a vegetable protein diet does not appear to cause this degree of kidney stress. When kidney disease patients switch from an animal protein diet to one based on soy, they excrete less protein in their urine. This indicates a lower risk of kidney failure.

# Q. Does soy play a role in the prevention of kidney stones?

**A.** Kidney stones, which are much more common in Western countries, can be formed when substances in urine, such as calcium, precipitate into stones. Animal protein contributes to kidney stones by causing more calcium to be excreted into the urine. In contrast, vegetable proteins, such as soy, do not cause as much calcium excretion, and thus reduce the risk of kidney stones. Studies show that vegetarians have half the risk of kidney stones as meat-eaters.

# Q. Can soy prevent gallstones?

**A.** Gallstones are round lumps of solid matter (often cholesterol) found in the gallbladder and sometimes in the bile ducts. Gallstones are fairly common, but only cause symptoms or complications in about 20 percent of cases. In addition, gallstones are two to three times more common in women than men.

Plant proteins in general and soy protein, in particular, have been shown to prevent gallstones. And soy may even shrink a gallstone after it has developed. Vegetarians, who often include frequent servings of soy in their diets, suffer from only half the gallstones of meat-eaters.

## Q. Is soy helpful for tinnitus?

A. Tinnitus is a hearing disorder that causes constant ringing, buzzing, whistling, hissing, or other noise heard in the ear. Although this condition is not well understood, it is believed that the acoustic nerve sends impulses to the brain as a result of messages sent within the head or ear itself—not as a response to environmental noise. Currently, there are very few treatments available for this frustrating condition.

Ipriflavone has been examined as a potential treatment for tinnitus. When nine tinnitus patients were given ipriflavone and seven others were given dummy pills for the sake of comparison, the ipriflavone-treated group showed promising results.

Another hearing disorder, called otosclerosis—a condition in which an overgrowth of bone prevents sound vibrations from passing into the inner ear and leads to deafness—might also be helped with ipriflavone treatment.

# Q. Are there any other health conditions that might benefit from soy?

**A.** Soy continues to be a hot topic of research. Researchers have conducted preliminary research suggesting that isoflavones might be a treatment for hereditary chronic nose-bleed syndrome and might play a role in the treatment of inflammatory and autoimmune disorders, as well.

# 8.

# How to Incorporate
# Soy Into Your Life

**B**y now it should be clear that finding ways to include more soy in your diet can reduce your risk of disease, whether you are concerned with heart disease, cancer, osteoporosis, or diabetes. This chapter will explain the various food choices you have for consuming soy and how to use soy supplements, if you prefer. Finally, minor side effects associated with soy will be discussed.

## Q. How much soy do I need to eat?

**A.** One should try to consume 25 to 45 mg of isoflavones each day. This is the amount that an average Japanese women eats, which makes it a good goal if you also want to have the enviably low rates of cancer and menopause symptoms seen in Japanese women. By way of comparison, the average American consumes less than 5 mg per day.

Clearly, we have a lot of room for improvement.

People who regularly incorporate soy foods into their lives (as little as one-and-a-half servings of soy daily) are afforded better cancer protection than those who only sporadically consume soy foods. Presumably, this holds true for the other health benefits of soy.

## Q. Does it matter which form of soy I eat?

**A.** Although taste preferences will probably be the main reason you choose one type of soy product over another, there are differences in isoflavone content that you may want to consider. For instance, tofu yogurt and soy hot dogs provide only one-tenth of the isoflavone content of whole soybeans, tofu, tempeh, and other less processed soy products. This is because other ingredients in these food products crowd out the soy. Even so, these soy products contain far more isoflavones than other plant sources (such as lentils, kidney beans, and garbanzo beans).

## Q. Can soybeans be eaten in their whole, unprocessed form?

**A.** Whole soybeans, a common item in Asian cuisine, provide the highest concentration of iso-flavones. Soybeans can be cooked and eaten in their fully mature, hardened form. In this way, they are prepared much the same as dried black beans, kidney beans, or garbanzo beans—that is, soaked in water for several hours and then simmered in plenty of water until tender.

Most mature soybeans are yellow, but brown and black varieties can also be found. However, soybeans are sometimes harvested while still in a green, immature stage. In this form they are very similar to green peas in a pod and have a firm, crisp texture. In Japan these immature soybeans are called *edamame*.

Whole soybeans can generally be found in health-food stores and Asian markets. The dried beans can be stored in an air-tight container for many months, however the fresh pods of soybeans should be kept in the refrigerator and used within two days or stored in the freezer for a few months.

## Q. Can you tell me more about tofu?

**A.** Tofu, a dietary staple throughout Asia, is made fresh daily in small tofu shops in Japan. Cooked whole soybeans are squeezed to yield a milklike liquid, which is then coagulated, much like cheese. In the United States, tofu is usually found prepackaged in the produce section of grocery stores or in Asian markets.

Freshly made tofu should be stored in the refrigerator in a container of water (with the water changed every day or so). However, tofu in aseptic packages can be stored on any kitchen shelf for much longer (refrigerate after opening). Tofu can also be kept in the freezer, which will change its texture to a firmer, chewy consistency.

Tofu is a great source of protein. In addition, tofu is rich in the B vitamins and iron. If calcium sulfate has been used in the preparation of tofu, it is also a source of calcium. Although tofu is 50-percent fat, it is usually used in dishes that overall are low-fat (such as vegetable stir-fry). And the fat that is in tofu is the healthier unsaturated fat and contains no cholesterol. Tofu is also very low in sodium, while its levels of phytoestrogens are quite high.

There are three common types of tofu. Firm tofu is the most dense, which makes it ideal in stir-fry dishes, on the barbecue, or in any recipe wherein you want it to retain its shape. Incidentally, firm tofu has the highest protein, fat, and calcium levels. Soft tofu is good for a dish that calls for mashing or blending the tofu. And the third, silken tofu, has a creamy texture and is very good pureéd. Silken tofu has the lowest fat content. Specialty low-fat tofu is also available.

# Q. Can soy milk be used to replace dairy milk?

**A.** Sure, soy milk is a great alternative to dairy milk, especially for anyone who is lactose intolerant. Like other soy foods, soy milk is a great source of protein, B vitamins, and iron. Many brands of soy milk have been fortified with additional nutrients to more closely approximate the nutritional profile of dairy milk. For example, many brands of soy milk contain added calcium, vitamin D, and vitamin $B_{12}$.

Soy milk is made by soaking and cooking whole soybeans and then expressing them into a rich, creamy liquid. Although a similar process is used to make tofu, soy milk is cooked longer. It is also sold in many grocery stores, health-food stores, and Asian markets. Although sometimes found freshly prepared in refrigerated sections of the store, it is more commonly sold in aseptic packages. These packages can be stored in the cupboard, but after opening they need to be refrigerated and used within a week. Soy milk is also sold in powdered forms, which should be stored in the refrigerator or freezer for best results. Many soy milks are flavored with vanilla, malt, barley, or cocoa, and some are even "lite," that is, made with reduced fat calories.

Although children can drink soy milk, infants should not be given soy milk because it doesn't contain all of the nutrients they require. Rather, infants should be fed breast milk (ideally), infant formula, or soy prepared into infant formula.

# Q. What is tempeh?

**A.** Tempeh is a traditional Indonesian food made with soy. It is made by combining whole soybeans with either rice or millet. A "starter" of a piece of tempeh from a previous batch or a mold culture is then added and all the ingredients are incubated for twenty-four hours. The final product is a hearty, chewy cake of beans that has a nutlike or even smoky flavor. The flavor of tempeh is sometimes compared to mushrooms.

Since tempeh is made from whole soybeans, it has all the nutrition of tofu and soy milk, but is also high in fiber. Tempeh can be grilled as a "burger" or added as chunks to other dishes.

Many stores carry tempeh in the frozen foods section. Kept frozen, it will last for many months, or about ten days in the refrigerator. Like other fermented products (such as cheese) a little mold on the surface can simply be cut off while the rest of the product is still edible.

## Q. Does tempeh have any advantages over tofu?

**A.** The fermentation process that turns soybeans into tempeh appears to make the isoflavones more usable and boost levels of several vitamins while reducing the fat content, as well. Another unique quality of tempeh is that this soy product appears to have antimicrobial activity that protects against and treats some types of diarrhea.

## Q. Is textured vegetable protein (TVP) made from soy?

**A.** It sure is. TVP, or textured soy protein as it is sometimes called, is made from soy flour. The flour is compressed until the protein fibers change in structure. TVP comes in a dehydrated form and is combined with boiling water before being added to a recipe, often in place of ground beef. TVP is high in protein, but very low in fat. In addition, TVP is also a good source of fiber. TVP has long been used by the military and schools to "extend" the amount of meat in such dishes as hamburgers, sloppy joes, and chili. But it can also used to completely replace meat in any of a number of dishes.

## Q. Are so-called meat analogs another potential source of soy?

**A.** Meat analogs are made from soy protein and mimic the look and taste of meat. They can be found in frozen, canned, or dried forms. Many are made from soy protein isolate, which is a high-protein, easily digested, low-fat food. Meat analogs are often surprisingly similar in taste and look to hamburgers, hot dogs, deli meats, and sausage, whereas dairy analogs mimic cheese, ice cream, and other dairy products.

## Q. Can soy flour be used as yet another source of soy?

**A.** Soy flour is made by roasting soybeans and then grinding them into a fine powder. Consequently, soy flour is a great source of protein, iron, calcium, and B vitamins. Soy flour can replace a portion of the regular flour in many recipes.

There are two types of soy flour. Regular soy

flour contains everything that is found in the natural soybean, while defatted soy flour has had the oil removed during processing. Both should be stored in the refrigerator or freezer.

## Q. What are okara and natto?

**A.** Okara is what is left behind after liquid has been extracted from soaked soybeans. Contrary to what it would seem, okara is light and fluffy. It is very high in both fiber and protein. Since it is very perishable in its fresh form, it is not widely available in any stores. However, okara is found in some premade vegetarian burgers.

Natto is a traditional Japanese food made by fermenting soybeans with a bacteria. Originally, this fermentation process took place in straw, resulting in a product with a faint strawlike flavor. Today, natto is made by incubating soybeans and bacteria in plastic bags, which results in a slightly different taste.

## Q. Does miso contain soy?

**A.** Miso is another fermented soy product. Soybeans and a grain (rice or barley), combined with salt and a species of beneficial bacteria, are aged for at least a year to produce a smooth paste with a salty taste. Traditionally, miso is used as a condiment or soup base.

Miso is found in health-food stores or Asian markets and should be stored in a covered container in the refrigerator. It is very salty, so keep in mind that a little goes a long way.

# Q. Is soy sauce a good source of soy?

**A.** Traditional soy sauce, called shoyu, is made by combining cooked soybeans, a grain, and a mold and allowing them to ferment in a salty brine for up to eighteen months. But the soy sauce used by most Americans is made by a very different, and inferior, process. This synthetic soy sauce is made by mixing defatted soybean meal with wheat, chemicals, caramel coloring, and corn syrup in a process lasting only a few days. As a result, the taste doesn't compare to traditional shoyu, and soy sauce is a poor source of isoflavones.

Shoyu (or tamari as it is sometimes called) can be found at Asian markets and some health-food stores. Bear in mind that shoyu and American soy sauce are very high in salt.

There has been some concern that the saltiness of

soy sauce may contribute to cancer after early laboratory studies showed disturbing results. However, follow-up studies in animals have not been able to demonstrate any risk, even at very high intakes of soy sauce. And some research shows that shoyu may prevent stomach cancer.

## Q. How healthy is soy oil?

**A.** The oil extracted from soybeans is low in saturated fat, contains no cholesterol, and is a source of omega-3 fatty acids (the kind found in fish that reduces the risk of heart disease). Soy oil accounts for as much as 75 percent of all the vegetable oil consumed by the average American. In fact, most oils that are labeled vegetable oil contain 100-percent soy oil. Soy oil has a light flavor and a high smoking point, which means that it doesn't smoke when you are frying at high temperatures.

## Q. What are my supplement options?

**A.** If the many soy foods described in this chapter don't interest you, or if you are looking for ways to really boost your soy intake, you should consider a soy supplement. Probably the most popular soy supplements are soy protein powders, which contain both soy protein and soy isoflavones. You simply mix the powder with juice, milk, or any other liquid. You could even add soy powder or soy flour into baked goods, like muffins or pancakes. Some soy powders come already premixed as shakes. There are also soy-based snack bars, but you'll pay a little extra for their convenience. Soy isoflavones also come in capsule or tablet form.

## Q. How much soy isoflavone should I take in supplement form?

**A.** As a general health insurance policy, following the example of the amount of soy isoflavones found in the average Asian diet is probably a great starting point. This amount, as mentioned earlier, is about 25 to 45 mg of isoflavones daily. Check the label of various supplements (such as powders, shakes, snack bars, or capsules) for the amount of isoflavones per serving, and adjust your intake accordingly.

Naturally, if you are using isoflavones for treatment instead of prevention, you'll need a higher intake of soy isoflavones. As a general rule, you may need about twice as much of the preventive dose. In other words, about 50 to 90 mg of isoflavones daily can be taken by women trying to control hot flashes, cholesterol levels, or other health concerns. Of course, a physician should also be consulted during the treatment of any disease.

## Q. What's the difference between soy foods and the soy in supplements?

**A.** Both soy foods and soy supplements have advantages unique to them. Soy foods are a healthy addition to any diet, and, by replacing higher fat and cholesterol-rich foods, can positively affect health.

However, the active ingredients of soy, in tablet or capsule form, are a convenient and hassle-free way to reap the benefits of soy—without making major dietary changes. They can increase your intake of isoflavones, but they cannot replace a healthy diet or instantly undo years of high-fat, low-nutrient food choices.

## Q. Are there any cautions to keep in mind when choosing soy foods or supplements?

**A.** If you are considering adding more soy foods into your diet there are just a few minor cautions. Suddenly eating soy at every meal can result in intestinal gas and discomfort. Instead, increase your intake gradually.

Compared with eggs, milk, and meat, soy has a slightly less than ideal ratio of amino acids. Fortunately, simply eating soy as part of a normal, varied diet compensates for the missing amino acids. In addition, soy may interfere with some mineral levels. Phytic acid in soy foods can bind in the intestines with minerals, such as calcium, iron, and zinc, preventing them from being absorbed. This, however, is rarely a problem. Increase your intakes of these minerals while taking soy.

Raw or unprocessed soybeans contain substances called protease inhibitors that interfere with the digestion of protein. During processing, up to 80 percent of protease inhibitors are deactivated. Given the fact that soybeans in the unprocessed form are tough and unappetizing, and so never eaten, protease inhibitors seem like an unimportant concern.

A very small percentage of people have allergies to soybeans. Although milk, peanut, or wheat allergies are much more common, some people do have allergies to soy, and this should be watched for.

# Conclusion

If you're a woman, no matter what your age or current health status, you've probably realized by now that soy has a lot to offer you. Soy-rich diets are strongly associated with a lower risk of hormone-related cancers, including breast and uterine cancers in women and prostate cancer in men. There is also a clear relationship between high-soy diets and lower blood cholesterol levels, which is in turn associated with a lower risk of heart disease. Hot flashes during menopause, in many women, occur with less frequency when supplementing with soy isoflavones.

Some women are even considering the use of soy isoflavones as a way to reduce the need for hormone replacement therapy. Soy isoflavones, and the related compound ipriflavone, also have roles in preventing and treating osteoporosis. As if that weren't enough, soy can provide important nutritional support for people with diabetes, kidney disease, gallstones, and tinnitus.

And don't forget the simple fact that soy is a

healthy addition to the diet, particularly as an alternative to protein from meat and dairy, which contain undesirable saturated fat and cholesterol. Soy is also very tasty. So whenever you eat soy foods, or take a soy supplement, know that you'll be getting a hefty dose of phytoestrogens and antioxidants to guard against a wide array of health conditions.

# Glossary

**Angiogenesis.** The process of forming new blood vessels in the body. Cancer cells use angiogenesis to grow and spread.

**Antioxidant.** A compound that neutralizes free radicals, which are associated with degenerative diseases such as cancer, heart disease, and premature aging.

**Coumestans.** One of the three main classes of phytoestrogens. Clover and some legumes are rich sources of coumestans.

**Daidzein.** One of the three types of isoflavones present in soy; it has estrogenlike activity.

**Endometriosis.** A health condition in which a woman experiences considerable pain, cramping, and heavy bleeding during menstruation.

**Estrogen.** One of the hormones produced by a woman's body that governs many body processes.

**Free radical.** A highly reactive compound that damages cell membranes and other cell components, contributing to degenerative diseases such as heart disease, cancer, premature aging, cataracts, and many other conditions. They are found in air pollution, tobacco smoke, some foods, pesticides, and ultraviolet radiation; they are also manufactured during normal body processes.

**Genistein.** One of the three types of isoflavones present in soy; it has estrogenlike activity.

**Ipriflavone.** A compound similar to isoflavone that prevents and treats osteoporosis.

**Isoflavone.** A compound in soy that has estrogen-like and antioxidant activity.

**Lignan.** One of the three main classes of phytoestrogens. Flaxseed oil and whole grains are rich sources of lignans.

**Phytic acid.** A component of soy and other high-fiber foods that has anti-cancer activity, though it may bind with minerals and inhibit their absorption.

**Phytoestrogen.** A plant compound that has estrogenlike activity in the body. Phytoestrogens are associated with a lower risk of menopause symptoms, breast cancer, heart disease, and osteoporosis.

**Phytosterol.** A compound in certain plants that has a similar structure to cholesterol, but is associated with a lower risk of heart disease and colon cancer.

**Protease inhibitors.** Compounds in soy that reduce the risk of cancer.

**Xenoestrogen.** Synthetic estrogens present in the environment that increase the risk of hormone-related cancers, such as breast, uterine, and prostate cancers.

# References

Adlercreutz H, Witold M, "Phyto-oestrogens and western diseases," *Ann Med* 29 (1997):95–120.

Adlercreutz H, et al., "Dietary phyto-oestrogens and the menopause in Japan," *Lancet* 339 (1992):1233.

Albertazzi P, Pansini F, Bonaccorsi G, et al., "The effect of dietary soy supplementation on hot flushes," *Ob Gyn* 91 (1998):6–11.

Anderson JW, Garner S, "Phytoestrogens and human function," *Nutr Today* 32(6) (1997):232–239.

Anderson JW, et al., "Meta-analysis of the effects of soy protein intake on serum lipids," *New Engl J Med* 333 (1995):276–282.

Barnes S, "Evolution of the health benefits of soy isoflavones," *Proc Soc Exp Biol Med* 21(1998): 386–392.

Bingham SA, Atkinson C, Liggins J, et al., "Phytoestrogens: where are we now?" *Br J Nutr* 79 (1998):393–406.

Brandi ML, "New treatment strategies: ipriflavone,

strontium, vitamin D metabolites and analogs," *Am J Med* 95(suppl 5A) (1993):69–74.

Cassidy A, et al., "Biological effects of a diet of soy protein rich in isoflavones on the menstrual cycle of premenopausal women," *Am J Clin Nutr* 60 (1994): 333–340.

Gennari C, Agnusdei D, Crepaldi G, et al., "Effect of ipriflavone—a synthetic derivative of natural iso-flavones—on bone mass loss in the early years after menopause," *Menopause* 5 (1998):5–15.

Goodman MT, Wilkens LR, Hankin JH, et al., "Association of soy and fiber consumption with the risk of endometrial cancer," *Am J Epidem* 146 (1997):294–306.

Knight D, Eden J, "A review of the clinical effects of phytoestrogens," *Ob Gyn* 87(5) (1996):897–903.

Kovás AB, "Efficacy of ipriflavone in the prevention and treatment of postmenopausal osteoporosis," *Agent Actions* 41 (1994):86–87.

Kurzer M, Xu X, "Dietary phytoestrogens," *Ann Rev Nutr* 17 (1997):353–381.

Lee HP, et al., "Dietary effects on breast-cancer risk in Singapore," *Lancet* 337 (1991):1197–1200.

Messina MJ, et al., "The role of soy products in reducing the risk of cancer," *J Natl Cancer Inst* 83(8) (1991):541–546.

Murkies AL, et al., "Dietary flour supplementation decreases post-menopausal hot flushes: Effect of soy and wheat," *Maturitas* 21(3) (1995):189–195.

Murkies A, Wilcox G, Davis S, "Phytoestrogens," *J Clin Endo Metab* 83(2) (1988):297–303.

Nagata C, Takatsuka N, Kurisu Y, et al., "Decreased serum total cholesterol concentration is associated with high intake of soy products in Japanese men and women," *J Nutr* 128 (1998):209–213.

Peterson G, et al., "Genistein inhibition of the growth of human breast cancer cells: independence from estrogen receptors and the multi-drug resistance gene," *Biochem Biophys Res Comm* 179(1) (1991):661–667.

Potter SM, "Overview of the proposed mechanisms for the hypocholesterolemic effect of soy," *J Nutr* 125(3 suppl) (1995):606–611.

Tham D, Gardner C, Haskell W, "Potential health benefits of dietary phytoestrogens: A review of the clinical, epidemiological, and mechanistic evidence," *J Clin Endo Metab* 83(7) (1998):2223–2235.

Wei H, et al., "Antioxidant and antipromotional effects of the soybean isoflavone genistein," *Proc Soc Exp Biol Med* 208 (1995):124–129.

# Suggested Readings

Gittleman A. *Super Nutrition for Menopause*. Garden City Park, NY: Avery Publishing Group, 1998.

Messina M and Messina V. *The Simple Soybean and Your Health*. Garden City Park, NY: Avery Publishing Group, 1994.

Somer E. *Nutrition for Women*. New York: Henry Holt, 1993.

# Index